TEACH ME YOUR ATTITUDE

By Patricia Desmond Vargo

ISBN: 1-4107-4183-4 (e-book)
ISBN: 1-4107-4182-6 (Paperback)

Library of Congress Control Number: 2003092279

This book is printed on acid free paper.

Printed in the United States of America
Bloomington, IN

1stBooks – rev. 04/04/03

INTRODUCTION

There were times during my life when I would passionately relay details of some experience to my mother. She would say, "Pat, you could write a book!" I thought that was a possibility, but I never dreamed it would be about her. Until three years ago her life seemed so simple, so uncomplicated.

Several months ago I began scripting events supporting her wonderful attitude. It gave me pleasure to reflect upon the joy she brings to others. In my perception, these events are true. Names have been changed to avoid obtaining endless permission. I am grateful for all. Even people who have hurt me played a part. They put me on the correct path to fulfill this mission. If real names were used for non-relatives, it is because they are considered family.

Thank you to my supportive family, co-workers, friends, and most importantly my sister who read this book first and lived this journey closer than anyone can imagine - Rita Claire Fitzsimmons, and, also, my brother, Paul Desmond.

Pat Vargo

Children - Kahil Gibran - from "The Prophet"

Your children are not your children

They are the sons and daughters of life's longing for itself.

They come through you, but not from you.

And though they are with you yet they belong not to you.

You may give them your love, but not your thoughts

For they have their own thoughts.

You may house their bodies, but not their souls

For their souls dwell in the house of tomorrow, which you cannot visit, not even in your dreams.

You may strive to be like them, but seek not to make them like you

For life goes not backward nor tarries with yesterday.

You are the bows from which your children as living arrows are sent forth.

The Archer sees the mark upon the path of the infinite and He bends you with His might that His arrows may go swift and far.

Let your bending in the Archer's Hand be for gladness

For even as He loves the arrow that flies

So He loves also the bow that is stable.

"When the student is ready the teacher will appear."

The teacher is a fifty-four year old woman and the student is her twenty-year old daughter. No wait-thirty-four years have passed. The teacher is an eighty-eight year old woman and her daughter is now fifty-four. The daughter felt cheated by her father's death thirty-four years ago. Her mother could have died the same year as her dad of hypertension. The doctor gave her mom pills to bring down the blood pressure. Her face was red and that brought her in for the checkup. She finished the prescription, but did not renew it because she was distracted by her grief. Subsequent

1

nosebleeds brought her back to the doctor. This time he sat her down and made sure she "got it". *These pills are to be renewed for life or you will die.*

Mom (Rita) has been a major player in her children and grandchildren's happiness. They are grateful for every second God allows her to live. They realize she must have fulfilled her earthly mission for herself and is spared to help them fulfill theirs.

Mom's ninety-eight year old sibling, Ruth, still refers to Rita as "my baby sister" and shared Mom's outlook early in life, earning her the nickname "Sunny". She was the only female cheerleader (There were two males.) at

St. Aloysius High School, Jersey City, New Jersey from 1927 to 1931. She and my Dad (Frank) met at a wedding they attended in 1935 when she was twenty-one and he was twenty-four. She took pride in the fact that he returned to his mother that evening claiming he met the woman he would some day marry. The fulfillment of this dream came on May 25, 1940. They had twenty-eight happy years together before their marriage ended with his death. Happy were July 4th and New Year's parties with the neighbors. There were church picnics and plays. They were present to their family and friends, cherished by all. They were like Ozzie and Harriet. We were blessed. Just when their responsibility to children ended and they could travel together it was over. My sister hid the pamphlets Dad left out on the table - the trip to Paris he and Mom would never have. She shoved them in a dining room drawer. Then we could agonize over it again when Mom would find them while looking for something else.

My sister and brother-in-law's three sons were babies, too young to remember their grandfather. There would be eight more grandchildren that he would never know, at least in this realm. Mom would bond with every one of them and they with her. Four have married and have children of their own. Mom adores every addition we've welcomed to our family. She's been blessed with seven great-grandchildren in five years. When you love, love, love and give energy to others-that is what comes back to you without intention or effort. It is just life's force and it is wonderful. We cannot control life or death, sun or rain, the Mets winning or losing, but we can love or not love each other. We can trust in God or be mad at Him. Rita trusts "God's will". God is never wrong. God is #1. That is our first lesson. Lesson #2 is that attitude is a choice.

My father died when I was twenty. I was in Bermuda vacationing with friends when the call came that I was to return to New Jersey because my father was not expected to live through the night. (The last greeting card I sent to my Dad said, "If all you need is rest and relaxation to get well… then how did you ever get sick in the first place?") I cannot explain the sense of impending doom I had felt prior to the phone call that changed my life. My friends rode motorbikes earlier that day, but I feared I would fall even though I mastered the vehicle. My friends went out in a rowboat not far from shore, but I was afraid I'd drown even though I could swim. There was no reasonable explanation for my anxiety until the call validated my premonition. The girl who told me I had to leave was the only one I did not know well. The other three, who were my friends, had eyes welled with tears. They helplessly witnessed me empty drawers into suitcases. My friends accompanied me to the airport in Bermuda. They were supportive. I cried all the way to Kennedy Airport. An actress, Paula Prentiss, came over to me on the flight to offer comfort. Then I met a cab driver who drove me to Port Authority Bus Terminal in New York City. When I shared my urgent circumstance he told me he flew home from his Army position overseas twenty years ago to say good-bye to his dying mother and that she is still alive today. His encouraging story gave me false hope, but I was grateful for it and his kind thoughts. My father died shortly before I arrived at the Jersey City hospital where I was born. It wasn't the funny story of how our next door neighbor missed "The Lone Ranger" driving Mom to the hospital the January night I was born or that I missed the snowstorm of '47 by one month. Alone in the room, I stared at him wondering if he was sleeping or dead. I approached my heartbroken mother in the corridor. When it was confirmed that he had passed on I thanked Mom for their good marriage and the example of love that I would cherish.

When we returned home and everyone made an attempt to end their exhaustion in sleep, I stayed awake wondering how we would cope emotionally as a family. My sister and brother were both married. I wanted to meet someone to marry and have children. If that dream became reality (and it did) this future husband and children of mine would never know my Dad. That was a difficult concept, one that was impossible to accept that night. Even though I was grateful for having a caring father for twenty years, I felt cheated. I wanted more time the way we were.

"But the souls of the just are in the hand of God, and
no torment shall touch them. They seemed, in the
view of the foolish, to be dead; and their passing away
was thought an affliction. But they are in peace."

Wisdom 3:1-3

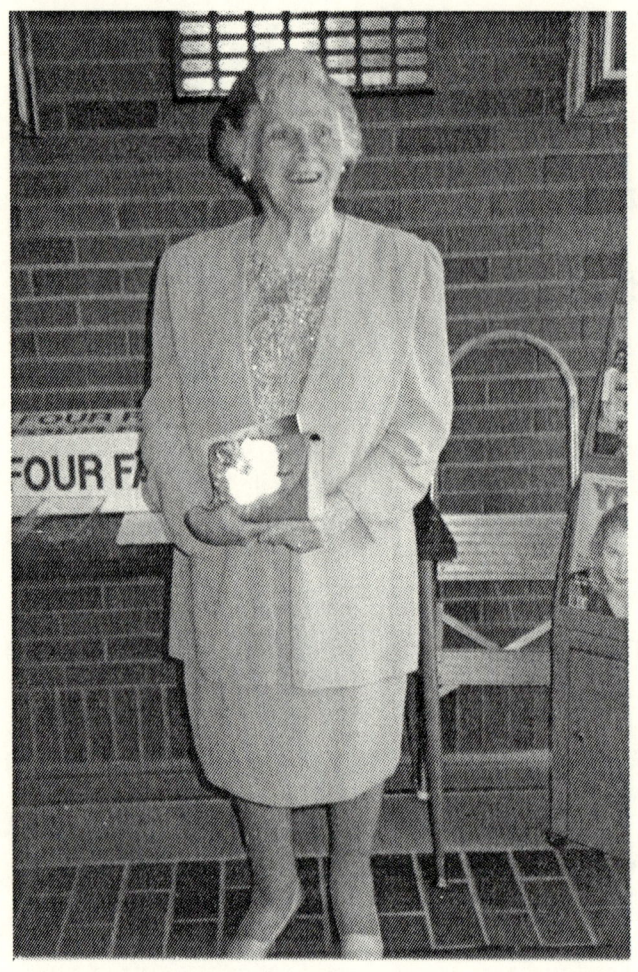

My mother is 88 years old now. She almost died Valentine's Day 2001 when she suffered a slight stroke. She jokes about it saying, "God's not ready for me yet and the devil won't have me." When the stroke happened, Mom had to give up her apartment and move into a healthcare facility where she could receive round-the-clock care. She did not want to live with a family member. Our family investigated facilities before she began rehabilitation. During this decision-making process Mom cried and admitted she was disappointed that she did not die. I knew she felt that way. I empathized. She was visually impaired from years of macular degeneration taking its toll. She had been unable to read for over three years. She can read a letter or a number if it was written very large in dark black marker. Now she was in a wheelchair because she could not walk. She used a walker before the stroke, but now her right

11

side was weak. My brother, Paul, watched helplessly as a cup of water slipped through Mom's failing grip of the right hand when she tried to drink by herself. As if that weren't enough to cope with, Mom was wearing diapers. Before the stroke she was totally continent. She had a sharp mind trapped in a body that would not function as it once had.

I knew she was having a pain in her leg the month before the stroke and I took her to the doctor. He suspected she had a blood clot in her leg and ordered an ultrasound. I took her to the hospital for the test. No blood clot was found. The reason is that the blood clot was in the opposite leg of the one that was tested by ultrasound. And so the stroke happened.

Mom was pushing her friend Beth in a wheelchair back to Beth's apartment following their senior Valentine party when she stumbled. Beth asked Mom if she was okay. Mom said although she felt lightheaded she thought she would be okay. It was a couple of hours from the time Mom fell down in her apartment until she dragged her half-paralyzed body along the carpet and up to the door where she could call for help. My sister, Rita Claire, and I both went to the hospital to meet the ambulance. After tests, it was confirmed she indeed suffered a stroke. After medication and initial treatment was implemented, Mom awaited room assignment. Rita Claire showed me that she had taken Mom's wedding ring off and I asked her to hold onto it. We kissed Mom goodnight and told her we would be back to visit the next day. She asked, "I'm staying here?" I replied "Mom, do you really think you can stand up and walk out of here with us?" She smiled and said, "No. See you tomorrow."

Aging macular degeneration is the thief that changes the beautiful world we see into distortion. It is described as the absence of central vision so that all that remains is vision from the corner of the eye (peripheral). Mom revisited an optometrist because she thought she needed new glasses when she was 76 years old. The day after we picked up the glasses she called to tell me there must have been some mistake because she still could not see well "The doctor gave me the wrong

14

glasses," she said. Something dropped inside me when she said that. What were the chances of the doctor giving her the wrong glasses? Not very good. I realized she had a visual problem that was not detected in the exam. The optometrist mentioned the start of cataracts and I hoped that it was a problem with a solution. I made an appointment with an ophthalmologist. He wanted Mom to see a retina specialist because he felt either she was not cooperating with the instructions, or she had a retina disease. Mom always tries to cooperate. Further testing confirmed the presence of the dry form of macular degeneration. The dry form was better to have than the wet because the deterioration came slowly. What we did not realize was that dry could turn to wet overnight with hemorrhage. Mom's disease was close to the center of the eye so the laser procedure was not recommended.

My cousin, Mark, called wanting Mom to see his wife, Ginger's, retina specialist in New York who reattached Ginger's retina, restoring some of her vision. I explained Mom's situation and said we would be happy to bring her into the city if there was hope. There was not. The New York doctor and Mom's New Jersey doctor attended medical school together. Mom was seventy-six with 20/20 vision, but that would change. Within 2 months she was 20/60. After two years the right eye would fail. The left would hold out allowing her to read another six years. At her senior complex, the Society for Prevention of Blindness encouraged her to use audio books and provided use of a machine. Unfortunately, the machine was not easy to operate. Mom spent early afternoons listening to tapes and CD's that my nephews bought her. Mom said listening to music from plays like "South Pacific" and "Oklahoma," and favorites like Frank Sinatra and the Lawrence Welk orchestra brought her to wonderful places in time and memory. It fixed her mood in gratitude. She did add alternative rock to her listening during the past year when my son, Jim, got a part time DJ position on a Sunday morning radio show in her listening area. All the young aides from the nursing

17

home saw another side of Mom and thought she was "cool" listening to U-2, Lenny Kravitz, and Linkin Park. At year's end she'd parrot Jim's remark, "I know which song is number one for the year, but you need to stay tuned because I'm not going to tell you!"

After Mom was bedridden with the stroke, I asked the neurologist the best scenario of when she may walk again. "Ten days would be the best, but your mother is not the best scenario. She's an eighty-seven-year-old woman who has severe arthritis and had serious health concerns before this stroke happened. She may recover to 99% of her prior stroke condition. That is possible," she reported. As she tested Mom I realized the weakness affecting her right side was extensive. Mom had only the slightest impairment of speech. She used a walker prior to the stroke. The right arm and leg would need to heal at the same time. She would need to exhaust herself in physical

19

therapy to regain her strength. The next stop was rehab.

The facility was one that housed both temporary and permanent patients. Mom would begin relentless therapy and we would meet two weeks later to discuss her progress. The doctors were amazed that Mom lived on her own independently as long as she had. She was highly functional in spite of her health concerns. She had been sleeping in her recliner at home. Lying down in a bed had become painful with her bent spine and then there was that problem of getting up again if she lay down.

The facility was clean and patients appeared well cared for, but it was still difficult to see Mom in a wheelchair in this setting. I wondered if I thought about this problem long enough I could come up with a solution of how she could live independently once again. After all, her friend Beth was in a wheelchair except Beth could see well and Mom could not. Beth could lift herself in the bathroom and into bed. Mom could not. She loved her senior residence and joked about its proximity to Higgins' Funeral Home and referred to it as "the last stop."

Mom felt living with us would put an unfair burden on us. The reality was she needed round the clock care and we all worked. We did not want her to be a prisoner isolated in our homes if the alternative was that she could attend activities and make friends to spend time with during the daytime. Mom's presence is a wonderful place for anyone to be.

I always trusted Mom's judgment and so I asked her, "Do you think you could live alone again?" Mom started to cry and admitted she needed assistance that was not available at her former senior home where she was so happy. She said she did not want to live with me, or my sister or brother, and asked if it were an option to remain in the facility. She shared again that she wished God had taken her before she would be faced with this difficult decision. She looked sad and my heart broke as I cried openly, unable to shield her from the emotion in my voice and the tears that she could see through her blindness.

Our family was relieved when a schedule for physical therapy was given to Mom. I had never seen Mom exercise and I was concerned by the weakness in her right side. What I did not realize initially was how much she would enjoy this exhilarating workout. Her therapists were devoted and often pulled her away from the breakfast table in an attempt to complete Medicare's expectation. After one week into therapy, I was wheeling Mom down the corridor when a doctor recognized her and introduced himself to me as Director of

23

Physical Therapy. He obtained a walker and asked Mom to stand and then walk using the walker while I pushed her empty wheelchair alongside. It was beyond belief that she was walking again. She walked about 25 feet sandwiched but unaided by the doctor and me. I couldn't wait to e-mail my sister and brother with this encouraging report. The therapy made this possible because she worked very hard to accomplish this goal. The therapists shared that Mom was a joy to work with-her attitude toward recovery was so positive. She could not understand why some patients would not try when these devoted therapists were giving them opportunities to become ambulatory and walk once again. "God helps those who help themselves" was Mom's motto when she wanted us to work hard toward a goal.

The awareness of the effects of osteoarthritis has been helpful in educating doctors and patients to take measures to either prevent or counteract effects of the gradual breakdown of cartilage between joints. However, the women who experienced menopause during the 1950's and 60's that are still living did not have the advantage of this awareness. Their bones - now 80 and 90 years old - suffered degenerative losses in the absence of hormone replacement therapy.

Nearing the millenium, Mom was incapacitated with sciatica and moved from the hospital emergency room into my family room for one month while she took strong painkillers and muscle relaxers waiting for the pain to subside. My sister, Rita Claire, and brother-in-law, John, took Mom to the orthopedist and he ordered a MRI. That became an ordeal. I got Mom there in a wheelchair and, while signing her in for the MRI, I overheard the technician mockingly laugh with the office helper that he had to do a lumbar spine MRI on an 85 year old woman "and didn't that sound like fun". There was a counter and glass window in the way of me grabbing him by the throat. Instead, I opened the glass window a tad and spoke in a tone loud enough for him (but too low for Mom) to hear, "You are speaking about my mother. You would not think this is so funny if it were your mother in pain." He froze like the proverbial deer caught in the headlights. I returned to Mom knowing I had him with a witness there. My energy was focused on getting her through this test. Shortly after Dr. Green started he came to me to say the test would be useless because Mom had a pessary (plastic device holding the bladder in place) obstructing the view of the spine. He recommended having it removed by a gynecologist or the hospital and then the MRI would give the information we needed. It was hours before we located her gynecologist. He

27

was nice enough to come to the hospital on his day off to do this for her. I returned several hours later to the MRI office and a different office shift was on. She told me she had no time to do my mother's test and that I would have to reschedule. Dr. Green was in earshot and walked over to us and said, "I will do her test now." Needless to say I never reported the prior unkind incident. Mom said she was not up to going to her Senior Residence Christmas party that same day. It was understandable that she was physically and emotionally exhausted. Yet I felt she needed that party for the soul-enriching experience it would be for her. Hey, I helplessly watched her suffer unbearable pain and, for that reason, would have to count that among the five most difficult days of my life. As we were driving home and she thanked me for guiding her through this day and if there was anything she could do for me. "Wait, stop right there. You know what you could do for me. Let me drop you off at the Christmas party and pick you up two hours later. Do it for me and for the friends who would like to spend time with you. Life has enough knocks. You completed a tough day today and need to celebrate." She went to the party and she had a great time.

Mom began pain management and was given two cortisone epidural shots a week apart in the spot the MRI indicated was troubled. I remember that at the first session the doctor asked if Mom had an irregular heartbeat. I said, "No," and made a silent prayer that he would not unveil an additional health problem. Mom struggled with the walker another two weeks until she felt an incredible improvement. Shortly after that time she was walking easily without her walker. Her neighbors remarked at her progress. It was months before she reported a pain in her ankle and we had X-rays to investigate whether or not it was a fracture. It was not; it was severe arthritis. As the doctor asked more questions we discovered Mom had been "the dancing queen" at her senior residence party. She admitted, "When I hear the music I can't help myself. I just have to dance!"

"Promise me you'll give faith a fighting
chance
and when you get the choice to sit it out or
dance -
I hope you dance…"
(Mark D. Sanders/Tia Sillers)

Lee Ann Womack . I Hope You Dance (2000)
I Hope You Dance
I hope you never lose your sense of wonder,
You get your fill to eat but always keep that
hunger, May you never take one single breath
for granted, God forbid love ever leave you
empty handed, I hope you still feel small when
you stand beside the ocean,
Whenever one door closes I hope one more
opens,
Promise me that you'll give faith a fighting
chance,
And when you get the choice to sit it our or
dance.
I hope you dance…..I hope you dance.

I hope you never fear those mountains in the
distance,
Never settle for the path of least resistance
Livin' might mean takin' chances but they're
worth takin',
Lovin' might be a mistake but it's worth
makin',
Don't let some hell bent heart leave you bitter,
When you come close to sellin' out
reconsider,
Give the heavens above more than just a
passing glance,
And when you get the choice to sit it our or
dance.
I hope you dance…..I hope you dance.
I hope you dance…..I hope you dance.
(Time is a wheel in constant motion always
rolling us along, Tell me who wants to look
back on their years and wonder where those
years have gone.)
I hope you still feel small when you stand
beside the ocean,
Whenever one door closes I hope one more
opens,

Promise me that you'll give faith a fighting
chance,
And when you get the choice to sit it out or
dance.
Dance…..I hope you dance.
I hope you dance…..I hope you dance.
I hope you dance…..I hope you dance..
(Time is a wheel in constant motion always
rolling us along
Tell me who wants to look back on their years
and wonder where those years have gone.

I know first-hand how difficult a decision it is to say my mother needs help-so much help that she cannot live alone anymore. We had been faced with a dilemma six years ago. Mom's hairdresser called Rita Claire to report that Mom's face was badly bruised. Mom admitted falling during the night. Due to her macular degeneration, Mom did not see how extensive her bruises were from hitting the corner of the end table. I threw the table out as if it were at fault. Mom had a CAT Scan to confirm it was not a stroke. Blood work indicated low potassium. She was given a supplement that corrected the imbalance. She never fell again.

Many times the decision to seek a health facility needs to be made at a time when we are suffering emotionally, as one would when a close family member suffers a stroke. Some people unfamiliar with the area involved may even have to shop for a good facility while visiting their ill parent and vacating the parent's former home. And if that weren't enough, there is the need to arrange a funeral without a death. A bed in a nursing facility is a limited commodity costing and earning thousands of dollars per month. It's big business. Under Medicaid, if you require a hospitalization for more than ten days, you lose your room unless you pay upward of $200 a day. To qualify for Medicaid, you need a financial net worth of less than $2000.

Patricia Desmond Vargo

You turn over your pension and social security and the state pays the remainder of the nearly $6500 monthly fee.

Rita Claire, Paul and I felt misled initially by the healthcare social placement manager. As Mom was about to be given placement for her room assignment, we were told that the lady in the room, Ginny, was really looking forward to meeting Mom. The social manager told us when Mom entered the room Ginny even came over to give her a hug. After Mom got settled in, had her phone installed, her new flex-a-bed and lift-chair delivered, and our pictures placed on the wall, we realized Ginny wasn't looking forward to Mom being her roommate. Ginny didn't know who she was

36

or where she was. We thought it was odd she did not have a phone. We realized the roommate was a gamble and, eventually, Ginny was moved to a wing where she could receive care that would not leave the bathroom unsanitary for another person. Mara was Mom's next roommate. She did not need a phone either because who are you going to call to constantly complain? When Mara woke up in the morning, the first words out of her mouth were, "I don't feel well." Then breakfast would come, "Oh no-not this crap." She was hopelessly waiting to go home which was never going to happen. Mom tried to explain, "Mara, we are home. This is our home." but Mara didn't get it. Mara never wanted to get out of bed so she could not tell day from night. It wasn't because she was mentally ill. It was pitiful - she didn't feel up to living. It was a sad choice. My siblings and I were determined to wait this one out, too, since Mom had a sunny half-room to which she'd grown accustomed. Ironically, even though Mom could not see someone's face she could enjoy the view of the flowers in the courtyard outside her window on the grounds.

Mara's depression deeply affected Mom and I explained to Mom that she needed to get herself out of the room as much as possible. This was the time Mom joined the garden coffee club, cooking class, choir and bingo. I told her if they have a luncheon getaway outside of the facility-sign up. Even if the outing is poorly attended, the bus driver was good company. Mom loved hearing nice stories about the workers' and residents' families. Eventually, Mara opted to move to a morgue-like location because she died inside a long time ago.

Mom's dining companions were wonderful. Carmella is mid 60's and asthmatic. She lost her memory for five years and then a talented geriatric physician medicated her back to normal. She was an angel of mercy to every roommate she had and took great joy in helping others.

Rosalie was soft spoken and understanding. She died a few months ago. Mom misses her but it is most difficult for Carmella since she and Rosalie were like sisters.

Mom's next roommate was Betty. The first day Betty was in the room, Mom's pocketbook disappeared. The aide found it in Betty's closet and she said, "That's mine". The aide said he would handle it and, as he removed papers with information on it that only Mom could identify, the case was closed. It was upsetting and Mom wondered if she should ask Betty's daughter if she had a pocketbook that was similar. I advised her not to-to just let it go. It never happened again. Betty was ninety-seven years old and had brain cancer – which explained the pocketbook incident. Betty was in a wheelchair, but had the eyes of an eagle and a quiet, positive outlook. She helped Mom by reading and identifying things Mom could not see. Mom helped retrieve things for Betty since Mom could walk around with her walker. Betty went to garden club with Mom and Mom jokingly added that nothing would be misplaced in her room if Betty were with her.

DIFFERENCE BETWEEN HEAVEN AND HELL

A man spoke with the Lord about heaven and hell.

The Lord said to the man, "Come, I will show you hell." They entered a room where a group of famished people sat around a huge pot of cooked stew. Everyone in the room was starving and desperate. Each person held a spoon that reached the pot, but each spoon had a handle so much longer than their own arms that it could not be used to get the stew into their own mouths. The suffering was terrible.

"Come, now I will show you heaven," the Lord said. They entered another room, identical to the first the big pot of stew, the group of people and the same long-handled spoons. But here everyone was happy and well-nourished.

"I don't understand," said the man. "Why is everyone happy here and miserable in the other room? Everything is the same."

"Here," said the Lord, "they have learned to feed each other."

One roommate Mom did transfer away from in rehab was Astrid. Astrid was ninety-two, obnoxious and outgoing. She said she had been unhappy in two other nursing homes, but we suspected she had been expelled for unacceptable behavior. She woke up screaming five times a night for no apparent reason and refused to use the call button to summon the nurse because that was not disruptive enough. The nurses came running, tending to her every need. When Astrid's daughter would call in the morning her mother would tell her "the help sucked and ignored her". Mom fought the urge to grab the phone out of her hand and tell the truth. Mom needed her energy to heal herself.

Astrid became a permanent resident and baited confrontation at every opportunity. She and Martha were like oil and water because Martha was outspoken and, being a resident for a long time, Mom said Martha thought she owned the place. Mom, being a sheltered person, brought up this dilemma at their monthly organized (griping session) meeting. Mom initiated her point by stating that the reputation of the healthcare facility was on the line if they were going to let two or three residents verbally abuse each other at social functions. Mom said, "I'm eighty-eight years old. I have never heard this language in my life and I'm not going to start now!" The staff acknowledged an awareness of this situation and promised that they would

45

carefully consider the negative effect it was causing others.

Meanwhile, judgmental Astrid continued to harass the residents calling them "animals" for not boarding the bus to go to St. Joseph's Church on Sunday. Mom said that maybe people weren't up to it. Astrid rebuffed Mom's excuse for others' behavior. Astrid told the residents daily that they shouldn't wear white shoes after Labor Day because her daughter said so. Mom asked, "Astrid, has your daughter been to the department stores lately? Because they are selling white shoes all year long." No. Astrid dictates what the residents wear and how they worship. It is ironic that someone who is so critical of

46

others' spiritual behavior is lacking a kind attitude herself. When Mom couldn't take it any more about the "animals" who didn't go to church she asked, "Astrid, did you go?" When Astrid said she did, Mom told her, "That is great! It is important that you got the opportunity to do what you wanted because we live in America and we are free to make choices. One of the choices I am making is that I am going to wear white shoes all year long." All the residents clapped.

I was looking forward to Mom's annual meeting at the healthcare facility where she was living because she had accomplished so much progress since the stroke one year before. Rita Claire and I work a few blocks from each other. I work in a furniture store as a service manager and Rita Claire is a secretary in the parochial school her sons attended. We had made plans to travel together to this meeting. The day before, I had taken Mom for her gynecological checkup. She was lethargic, claiming to have caught the stomach virus so many residents at the nursing home had. The following day Mom's doctor called me because she was admitting Mom to the hospital emergency room. Mom had unexplained fever and abdominal pain the doctor suspected was an obstruction. When I reached the hospital I was surprised to see her body shaking. I asked if she was having a heart attack and the nurse explained that her heartbeat was too rapid. They were giving her medication to slow it down.

The culprits were gallstones and although the heart stabilized and fever broke, her life was endangered by plummeting blood pressure. It improved during my evening visit, but dropped later that evening. Dr. Shikha called me at 1:40 am to say that Mom was being moved to the Intensive Care Unit because her blood pressure dropped alarmingly low and her liver enzymes were high. I remember the word "septic" and a reminder that age was not on our side. I would later learn she had blood poisoning, e-coli, and jaundice and her white count rose to 40,000. It was ironic to think that after 34 years of hypertension, we could lose her to low blood pressure.

I showered to wake myself up and returned to the hospital to tell her I wanted her to survive this. The nurse shared that Mom wasn't happy that I was called in the middle of the night (even if her life was on the line). I showed the nurse the title of this book because carrying the manuscript brought me comfort. I started writing it months ago and had not told Mom yet. The nurse said she admired

Mom's strength in the face of this crisis. I told her I came as soon as I could to make sure that Mom doesn't give up on her health. The nurses and doctors questioned the living will and I explained my sister initiated it so that Mom would not be forced to live if she had a massive stroke causing major incapacitation. This was an infection we hoped she would beat. She was walking around yesterday not that anyone would guess that by the looks of her. I told the nurse I wanted Mom to recover totally from this infection and then some time in the future to die in her sleep-but not tonight.

"Ask and you will receive. Seek and you will find. Knock, and it will be opened to you."

Matthew 7:7

When I entered intensive care I saw Mom in Room 4 and said, "Hi!" "Pat, Is that you? I can't believe they called you in the middle of the night," she said. I replied, "You are going to fight this, right?" She said, "Yes!" The nurse with her introduced herself as Tanya and explained she was setting up Mom's I.V. and that if I went to the waiting area she would come for me as soon as she completed the task (of getting this blood pressure raising drug in the works). I waited for twenty minutes before she led me back to Mom telling me Mom looked very excited to see me. I promised I would allow Mom to rest in her failing condition. Mom was sleeping when I entered. Actually she was snoring. I closed my eyes and meditated in prayer with the assurance that the noise of her breathing was telling me she is still alive. A half-hour later a man checked her vital signs and whispered excitedly that her blood pressure was coming back up nicely and the doctor would be happy with this report. I told Tanya I was going home to bed fifteen minutes away and she promised to call me if there was any change. I left the hospital at 3:45 a.m. and slept until 6:30. While my husband, Bob, and I were having coffee Dr. Arnold called. He said he wanted to remove Mom's blockage despite the risk she may not survive the procedure. Her kidneys were now failing. I asked what her chances were if he did not do it and he agreed that she had no chance. I told him to go for it, get a renal expert in for the kidneys and that Mom had two sisters, Ruth ninety-eight years old, and Gert at ninety-three years, who had amazed doctors in the past.

My Uncle Bill died in 1966 of pulmonary disease. He was fifty-seven years old and a heavy smoker. Bill was always the life of the party and we remember laughter whenever he was around. His four sisters affectionately referred to him as a "rascal."

My mother's sister, Mary, died four years ago at ninety-three years of age. She suffered dementia in her later years, but had a good life until then. Her faithful daughter, (my cousin) Ruth Ann, visited her almost every day. She misses the times with her mother before illness took over. My Aunt Ruth, who did not have children, is now like her mother. Mary lost her son, Gerard, to cancer when he was fifty-four and she was eighty. Her older son, Richard, was widowed unexpectedly a year ago. Natalie was his life.

Gert is ninety-three. She had back surgery two months ago to fuse bones after a fall off a stepstool. Her children MJ and Mark carefully weighed the surgery option. They found a talented doctor who pretended Gert was his mom during the decision making process. I tried to give blood for Aunt Gert prior to her surgery and failed by a tenth of a point. Fortunately she did not need it. Despite a serious bout of bronchitis after the surgery, she survived the procedure.

Ruth, at ninety-eight, suffered heart disease fifteen years ago. Then five years ago she had colon cancer (which my Mom survived at age seventy-three). The doctors did laser but a team consulted and determined long term plans for Ruth must include surgery that was successful. Then, four years ago, feisty Ruth lost her glove on a banister and tumbled down fourteen cement church steps. My cousin, MJ, was horrified when she turned Ruth over and saw her badly bruised face. There were no broken bones. I told my friend, Peggy, possibly Ruth's winter coat protected her. Peg said it sounded more like a team of angels with Ruth's deceased husband, Vincent, holding a net under her as she went down. I hope that all the doctors that have saved my Aunt Ruth over the years are doing as well as she is.

"Angel of God, my guardian dear to whom God's love commits me here. Ever this day be at my side - to light and guide - to rule and guard. Amen."

I called my brother and sister to give them Dr. Arnold's update. Rita Claire was coming out of the shower and Paul was in transit to his job in New York. I got through to my aunts for prayers. I broke down on Peggy's voice mail and then hated myself for it since she was a teacher just starting her day.

My twenty-four-year-old daughter, Danielle, and I went to the hospital at 9 a.m. and were pleasantly surprised to hear Mom say she slept well. The renal expert, Dr. Alaire, and the anesthesiologist briefed us. Rita Claire arrived with Father George who gave Mom the Roman Catholic last rights. We all prayed together with Mom holding hands. Mom said she was in God's hands and was accepting His will for her. Mom's lack of fear put us at ease. When Father George sensed a teachable moment for all of us, he asked Mom to share her life secret with her granddaughter, Danielle. Mom shared she had total trust in God and a wonderful family for which she was grateful. We all smiled at each other and felt peace in our hearts.

"Though I walk through the valley of the shadow of death, I will not fear, Thou art with me."(King David)

Psalm 23:4

It was three hours before Dr. Arnold returned to us as happy as one can be when he just saved someone's life. He told us he removed the blockage that was a stone in the liver and that he put a shunt in to drain the infected bile. He said he would give her a few days to heal and then go back in for the gallstones. The following day the surgeon would remove the gall bladder or this would happen again. When Mom returned a short time later she said she was awake for the procedure although she felt no pain. She said four or five doctors surrounded her and got the feeling they were pleased with what transpired. She was right. In the hands of God Mom was powerful.

"Dismiss all anxiety from your minds. Present your needs to God in every form of prayer and in petitions full of gratitude. Then God's own peace, which is beyond all understanding will stand guard over your hearts and minds."

Philippians 4:6

Mom was a great teacher of spirituality in our formative years as she guided us. We were taught prayers as soon as we could speak. We were reminded to be grateful before it was a proven health asset to feel that way. Mom's upbringing was strict. As Roman Catholics, they were quizzed about the Sunday gospel by their father at the dinner table. It taught them to listen and not daydream when God was speaking to them through scripture. They had their share of hardship. When Mom was eleven years old, she lost her thirteen-year-old brother, Jim, to rheumatic heart. Mom missed her brother. Watching her parents suffer this loss was difficult. They prayed for strength. They needed strength when I was five years old. I do not remember, but Rita Claire was twelve and saw our Dad cry. The day before Mom's parents were to celebrate fifty years of marriage, her father suffered a massive heart attack and died. Instead of a happy anniversary party there was a somber funeral. The timing of the special anniversary and absence of illness made his unexpected passing devastating. The undertaker told my grandmother it would be thirteen years before there was room in Papa's grave for her. She said, "I'll wait." She died fourteen years later.

1 Thessalonians 4: 13-18
"We do not want you to be unaware, brothers and sisters, about those who have fallen asleep, so that you may not grieve like the rest, who have no hope. For if we believe that Jesus died and rose, so too will God, through Jesus, bring with him those who have fallen asleep."

Faith was more than comfort during tragedy. It was a confidence that God would sort out situations even if they did not make sense to them. Mom's generation did not question their religion. They accepted and lived good lives. My aunts were all faith-filled and often turned to prayer and novena devotions for favors. One incident that stands out was when my sixty-year old cousin, MJ, was told she had lung cancer by a doctor reading her X-ray. Her mother, Gert, my mother, Rita, and Aunt Ruth went into novena mode and prayed incessantly for days like cloistered nuns. When my cousin went for her biopsy the doctor admitted that the tests were confusing the experts. The bottom line was that my cousin had a serious infection, but not lung cancer. Some would think this doctor was not competent. Our family was thankful MJ was given this second chance at life. To me it was nothing short of a miracle.

Mom did her job of surviving the procedure removing the blockage. Supposedly the worst was over.

Next, Dr. Arnold removed the gallstones. He waited five days because she was very ill. She had oodles of stones and, to his credit, follow-up tests confirmed that he got them all in one shot. The next day the surgeon went in to remove the gall bladder. We threw the word "laser" around inviting a less-invasive procedure into our thoughts. It did not fit Mom's fate. The gall bladder was inflamed and infected. There was no smooth sailing. We were high on Mom's initial survival when the doctors were skeptical. They did get a glimpse of our perception of Mom after the gallstones were bypassed. They knew she was strong in spite of several health concerns. They told her she was doing well, but she knew better. Despite her optimism, she's a realist who said, "I wish I were doing as well as the doctors claim. It's not happening. I don't feel like eating; I feel full. A doctor or nurse accused me of eating too many ice chips."

"Let me get this straight," I asked. "You can't have ice chips for your dry mouth, but you have unlimited push-button use of morphine literally at your fingertips?"

We sat on this discouragement for six days. Rita Claire and Paul wanted accountability. Tests were ordered to validate Mom's take on this. Now she had a blockage similar to the one with which she entered the emergency room.

In procedure #1, Dr. Arnold removed the blockage by inserting a stent.

In procedure #2, Dr. Arnold removed the gallstones in the bile duct and other multiple stones.

In procedure #3, the gall bladder was removed. When clipping off the area where the gall bladder used to be, one clip obstructs the bile duct causing the abdomen to accept what it meant to excrete.

In procedure #4, Dr. Arnold repeats procedure #1, but now, in addition to septic shock, Mom is breathing through a ventilator, has a temperature of 101 degrees, pneumonia, peritonitis, and blood sugar levels roller-coasting highs and lows, hasn't eaten in a week and feels guilty going into this procedure having been scolded for eating too many ice chips.

When we went to the recovery room, Rita Claire and I were relieved. Mom couldn't talk. Even her good attitude had to be questioning the "living will" she assumed would protect her from invasive extraordinary measures. This wasn't supposed to be that. We figured we were in trouble when Mom was moving her lips. We all needed time. Mom needed time to heal and gain her strength. Rita Claire and I needed time to digest all that had transpired. We made a decision to spend $212 a day to hold Mom's half-room at the nursing home.

If all went on schedule, Mom would have been back there now participating in choir for Easter. No! Instead she's fighting for her life once again because a clip threatens her lifeline. She always wants to please us so we use that as a ploy to our advantage. We'd surrender her to a massive stroke. That would be out of our control. It was beyond belief that while in an accredited hospital, under the scrutiny of twelve to twenty savvy doctors, that eighty-eight years of life, having survived all that she had, could be snuffed out because they did not track the clips.

"First do no harm."
A Doctor's Hippocratic Oath."

Patricia Desmond Vargo

Our Good Friday started a few weeks early this year. We want her at our dining table with a Dewar's on the rocks in her hand. We want to hear her say for the billionth time, "Isn't it nice we're all here together?"

Her mouth is parched - so uncomfortably dry. What is she thinking as she suffers? We're relieved to learn there's an explanation with a game plan. She beat the odds only to have them stacked against her once again.

Meanwhile, the prayer chain in Union is disrupted when ninety-eight year old, Aunt Ruth, suffers a heart attack. Caretaker, Christine, drives Aunt Gert to St. Elizabeth's

Hospital to wait for the ambulance. When it did not come, they returned home to find a medical team working feverishly on Ruth in the ambulance outside their home. After they succeed, deliver Ruth to the hospital and she stabilizes, the doctor says she needs twenty-four hour care and ninety-three year old, Aunt Gert, says, "I'm with her," as she tried to bury her cane behind her chair. Gert sees the humor in her offer. Last Tuesday, Gert almost lost both sisters on the same day. Gert said that Ruth's request for her first post-trauma meal was a cup of tea with a graham cracker. At ninety-eight, Ruth still has her own teeth.

Mom's been sleeping for three days since procedure #4. I begin Friday with early morning Mass and reached the office at 9:00 a.m. I worked for two hours before my 11:00 a.m. visit with Mom at the hospital, which, luckily, is only a five-minute drive. She was still sleeping, but opened her eyes for a few seconds trying to speak. Attached to a ventilator with a tube running down her throat, it is impossible for her to speak. She also has a tube inserted in her nose leading to the abdomen emptying gallons of bile that has infected her insides with peritonitis. She is sedated. Mom rests and heals and "weeps" both through her skin and in the way her body trembles. I know her movements so well.

I returned to work and called Rita Claire and Paul with updates. Rita Claire is going to the hospital at 4:00 p.m. Paul becomes confrontational about Mom's unnecessary suffering. He was not happy with the way she looked last weekend. Why did they always wait so long for follow-up tests? I agreed it is unfair, but I want us to focus our positive energy in prayer for her recovery. He questions me about her doctors so I offer to fax him their business cards with a brief history of what transpired including drawings that Dr. Arnold sketched of the position of the troublesome clip left near the bile duct.

Discussing legal aspects while Mom is fighting for her life exhausts me. I tell him I promise I'll discuss it after she's better. Her need for our prayers is urgent. It is a

73

disappointment to see her still on the ventilator at 4:00 p.m. Rita Claire and I tell her that it's Friday at 4:00 p.m. Mom always wants to know what time it is. We discuss Paul's reactions and hope Mom will be better when he comes the next day. I greeted Paul and his wife, Loretta, in the hallway on Saturday to warn them that Mom does not look good even though her vital signs are holding. Paul said he spoke to an attorney who advised him to take a picture of Mom. I asked him not to take the picture and he complied.

Dr. Arnold took the time to draw for us illustrations of Mom's situation. He called his mentor at Georgetown University to discuss Mom's case. He advised us to focus on Mom's recovery now and do what our conscience tells us later. He shares that his parents lost his infant sister in the 1950's due to a doctor's error. When people asked his mother why she did not sue, she said, "It will not bring her back."

He told us he was confident in the procedure he planned to open Mom's duct. She needed time to heal before attempting this; she had been through so much. He did not think she could survive surgery, and that's what his mentor confirmed in their recent phone conversation.

We left because Mom was getting frustrated trying to communicate. We told her we loved her and would see her later. She had to have questions. I told her she was right when a week ago she said she was not better. I told her that Dr. Arnold found a clip in her bile duct from the surgery and inserted a tube through her nose to relieve the bile fluid infecting her abdomen. I asked her if she could feel the relief and she nodded. When I told her that she would be O.K. she flipped her hands and rolled her eyes in a "How much more can I take?" response. She had a right to be angry.

Paul appeared calmer after Dr. Arnold walked us through his plan to balloon out the duct avoiding surgery altogether. Paul left his thirty-year career with Fiduciary Trust one year before losing several former coworkers and close friends on September 11th. He works in the financial district with the devastation that remains in his face. His wife, Loretta, a producer at NBC, was given cipro in the first anthrax incident. How can Paul expect life to be fair to his beloved mother? We all learned on September 11th how life can change in a moment. Paul looks the same on the outside, but he takes no one for granted. He says that when he looks at the Ground Zero site, he still sees the faces of all his lost friends.

Mom was taken off the ventilator mid-weekend. I was happy when I called Sunday morning to learn she was able to remain off it throughout the night. They prepped and then took her for an abdomen CAT scan.

Rita Claire came shortly after that. We were thumbs-upping each other and blessing ourselves in thanksgiving as the on-duty surgeon disconnected a several foot tube through the nose.

The nurse told Mom that while she was sleeping her roommate's daughter came to see her. Mom said, "Tell me again about Betty's daughter." I told Mom she'd be returning to the nursing home (Bentley) soon. She laughed with a tad of sarcasm. Rita Claire and I made eye contact. Hearing Mom's laughter after twelve days of hell - priceless!

I asked Mom if she remembered me telling her why this all happened. She did not. I repeated the story determined to keep her in the loop. She waited about ten seconds and said, "Tell me again about what happened." It wasn't time to say that Dr. Arnold's game plan is to balloon open the duct. He is confident that he can perform this procedure and that it will be successful.

The following day I was pleased to see Mom out of bed sitting in a chair. Bill Kanzler was there. Bill and his wife, Diane, are the best friends of Rita Claire and John - their homes have been back to back for thirty-five years. A retired business owner, Bill spends his mornings and afternoons doing the spiritual and corporal works of mercy. I see him assisting at 8:30 a.m. Mass every morning. He visits Mom and a resident named Mary on Wednesdays at the Bentley. He even came to the emergency room when he noticed that Mom's walker was in her room and she wasn't. When he left the emergency room after his visit he said, "Mrs. Desmond, the good news is that I'm leaving. The bad news is that I'll be back again tomorrow to visit."

Mom said Bill is such a comfort to her. She says that after he leaves she continues to replay the pleasant exchange in her head.

Rita Claire and John go to visit between my noon and evening visits. Mom looked good to them. Rita Claire reiterated the nurses pushing Mom to take more fluids and food than she felt able to consume. She took a little - they wanted more. They wanted Mom to improve to the next level. Mom needed more time.

By the time I return at 7:30 p.m., Mom is in pain saying, "God, help me. I've been ringing for the nurse a long time. Nobody comes." She wants ice chips. I get them and let the nursing staff know I'm unhappy with their lack of response. I asked, "Where do you go when you can't get help in intensive care?" I ask them to keep in mind an error put her there saying, "God, help me," instead of being at her assisted living home evening bingo game.

Mom tells me she feels badly she's "spoiling" our Easter. I told her, "Mom, God is helping you. He's receiving relentless prayers on your behalf. You are not spoiling our Easter. Your presence is our resurrection.

I had told Bob that prior to the last three years I was losing Mom piece by piece when she lost most of her vision. It hurts to watch her suffer. I console myself and her knowing that every pain I feel in my gut in love for her is suffering being lifted from her shoulders. I believe that when my brother-in-law, John, prays the rosary over with Mom in his evening visits, he is Christ's instrument carrying her cross for a few steps. Good Friday is not only 1969 years ago on Calvary. It is today in CentraState Hospital in Freehold, New Jersey, the town Bruce Springsteen has in his heart when he sings, "My Hometown."

I the Lord of snow and rain
I have borne my people's pain
I have wept for love of them
They turn away.

I will break their hearts of stone
Give them hearts for love alone
I will bring my light to them
Whom shall I send?

Here I am Lord
Is it I Lord
I have heard you calling in the night
I will go Lord if you lead my
I will hold your people in my heart.

Isaiah 6

When I went to work I offered to work on my day off to make up hours I have flexed to be present with Mom at crisis times at the hospital. My boss says I can do whatever I want to do. I feel relieved. I thank God I am not still working for Gary as I did when Mom had sciatica.

I was on break in the lunchroom on my last work position when Danielle called to say, "Grandma called. She's in pain. She said she can't walk." I put in an emergency call to Mom's physician and awaited his instructions leaving my work number. Since the phone in the lunchroom was not dependable I opted to wait for the call at my desk and spend the

85

remainder of my break reading. Gary came over and asked what I was reading in a tone that suggested sincerity. After I told him and he realized it wasn't technically related to my job, he vomited verbal assault against pleasure reading at my desk even though it was unpaid time. I thought about sharing my personal dilemma. Then I realized it would not have mattered. If his own mother called in pain he might tell her it was not a good time for him since he had such an important work position. If I told him my elderly mother was alone and frightened with pain, Gary might say, "And this affects me how?" I could not sell myself out to beat up tactics and putting family last. Choosing between Gary's tantrums and

Mom's needs was the easiest decision I ever made.

Dr. Shikha called me at work and I sensed bad news was coming from the tone of her voice. A doppler study unveiled a free-floating blood clot in Mom's left leg. That could travel and be fatal. The first option was heparin, but it was risky for an eighty-eight year old with bleeding potential. Option two was inserting a filter in the vein. That was a go - the sooner, the better.

Mom was apprehensive, "Another procedure?" I explained it would help leg pain. I told her the Press published an article on macular degeneration in today's paper and she asked, "Pat, when do you get time to read the paper?" I told her we all make time for what is important to us.

After the procedure, Rita Claire called sounding optimistic, "She is tired, but she is better." Mom was wonderful in my evening visit. She relaxed more peacefully than she had in weeks. I put moisturizer cream on her face. Then I fed her ice cream and sang with the late Jim Croce, "Every time I tried to tell you the words just came out wrong - so I had to say I love you in a song." The next time the verse came around she sang it with me. I told her I have three more words for you besides "I love you." I said, "You made it!" She smiled and said, "I made it." She looked joyful. The tug of war with the other realm was in our favor for now and on our side of the line. I pulled her a few inches closer - just to be on the safe side.

Rita Claire and I drove up to Union to see Aunt Ruth. She was home from the hospital, but the news was not good. She was given the prognosis of one week to live. We could not tell Mom who was fighting for her own life and too ill to accept this news. Hospice was involved in Aunt Ruth's release.

Ruth knew Rita Claire and I were there. Ruth Ann and MJ were there as well as Aunt Gert and her caretaker, Christine. Aunt Ruth joined in our conversations. When we were leaving she said, "Your mother's alright?" We said. "Yes." She told us, "I could write a book." We knew this was it and we were blessed that it was a peaceful and loving encounter.

Meanwhile Mom had a horrible day. When I went in the morning she was calling out for help. "Pat, please help me." When asked what she wanted help with she could not respond. Peggy stopped in the afternoon. Bill came later and watched helplessly. Later John went and saw the same psychotic display. When Rita Claire told him Danielle and Todd were on their way to visit he advised that they should not go. I called them on their cell phone and requested an about face. I called Dr. Shikha and learned Mom had been given adovan at 11:45 p.m. last night and it was known to make people crazy. It defied belief that this was administered in direct contradiction to the doctor's orders. "What part of, We do not want our mother fed psychotic drugs don't you get?" I called the floor nurse and complained. I begged, "Get my mother off that floor as fast as you can. You can keep your $35,000 bed. I want a bed my mother can be wheeled away from. Also, you know what you can do with your $1200 a bottle protein IV. I want my mother to eat real food--even one spoonful would be a start."

Danielle and I visited Mom in her new room on another floor and she looked better. She was tired, but peaceful in the absence of that ICU tension. We left soon after because Mom needed her rest. Physical therapy was scheduled for tomorrow. We lost the battle of Thursday, but not the war. If prayers were ammunition we would be on to victory soon, but we weren't there yet.

My jubilation at seeing Mom detached from life support and breathing on her own was short-lived. All vital signs were strong. Reinforcements were in place to keep infection and diabetes complications at bay. She needed to eat - to consume protein liquids - but desire wasn't there. We know Mom suffers from back pain. However, now that sedation has worn off, the discomfort was more than she could bear. She said, "God, help me," repeatedly. I asked the staff to reinforce Mom through this critical transition.

The following morning I reached for a pair of jeans that were too tight last month. With half of my insides gone, I knew that they would fit now. I left work on my lunch break. Mom told me that she had been calling out during the night and that the nurse told her that she was not the only patient there. My exterior remained calm for her benefit. I could feel my heart pounding, raging with anger that the nurse did not instead say, "Hang in, Rita, honey. I'll be back," like the other caretakers did. I later learned the young nurse's other patient was a handsome young man.

Mom wanted ice chips, so I ran out to get them asking which nurse was assigned to Mom today. Then I found myself defensively explaining that even though Mom is saying, "God, help me," every fifteen seconds, she has to be in excruciating pain to behave this way.

95

She is not a complainer like me. One nurse asked me to tell the nurse manager of the lack of staff response Mom was experiencing. I asked her to report it for me. She did.

Mom asked if she should give up in her agony. I said, "Fight, fight, fight," as I took three tae-kwon-do punches and step movements. She smiled. I read the poem, "Footprints," from my memory. Mom smiled and said, "That will give me something nice to think about." She closed her eyes to rest.

FOOTPRINTS

One night a woman had a dream. She dreamed she was walking along the beach with the Lord. Across the sky flashed scenes from her life. For each scene she noticed two sets of footprints in the sand, one belonged to her and the other to the Lord.

When the last scene of her l life flashed before her she looked back at the footprints in the sand. She noticed that many times along the path of her life there was only one set of footprints. She also noticed that it happened at the very lowest and saddest times of her life.

This really bothered her and she questioned the Lord about it.

"Lord, you said that once I decided to follow you, you'd walk with me all the way. But I have noticed that during the most troublesome times of my life there is only one set of footprints.

I don't understand why when I needed you most you would leave me."

The Lord replied, "My precious child, I love you and I would never leave you. During your times of trial and suffering when you see only one set of footprints, it was then that I carried you."

I returned to work and called Rita Claire to inform her of what had transpired. She was leaving work to resume our "watch" of Mom in her despair.

In my fragile state, I lost it with a customer. I said something about my mother's situation that was unprofessional and inappropriate. She went in for the kill asking for the owner. My boss acknowledged my error and told her he would "take care of it." Sensing my remorse he knew that was already done. Not a particularly demonstrative guy, he gives me a hug. We agree I need the rest of the week off and make Mom's recovery my job. I'm supposed to be his troubleshooter. Instead I create problems for him in my wake.

Seven years of prior Nordstrom "no problem" customer service and "through these doors walk the most courteous people in the world" had gone out the window. Today I needed empathy. Today I needed to be the customer.

My boss suggested I speak with, first, the floor nurse manager (as the staff member suggested) and, second, to Mrs. Reed, the patient representative. He thought I was spending too much time at the hospital and needed to be home more. Yet, when his twenty-four year old son was recently hospitalized, he flew across the country to be present and supportive to his first-born. I pretend to be going home but, instead, I returned to the hospital. Rita Claire was with Mom and frustrated with Mom's uncharacteristic mental attitude. When I reviewed my boss's advice to us, she told me she already had spoken to Mrs. Reed on the way into the hospital. Mrs. Reed had been Rita Claire and John's next-door neighbor when they moved into their house.

When I spoke to the floor nurse supervisor I summarized the four procedures Mom endured and our frustration that we weren't getting the staff support we had enjoyed until this time. She said she felt the nurse in question had potential but was insensitive. She would address it. Her eyes showed sincerity and I felt well received. I also shared what Mom said, "Those nurses must think that I am awful." I told her, "My mother did not come this far to be pushed around. We need you on our side. She's giving up."

I returned to Rita Claire and told her that when Mom said, "Maybe it's time for me to die." I disagreed and briefly presented the logic of all she overcame and then verbally pushed her back in the ring. I stood in the corner of the ring rooting. We would keep Paul informed tempering his already wits-end position. Our encouragement to Mom was relentless. "May the best woman win." Mom appeared battered as a fallen boxer having collapsed with bruises from revolving-door blood transfusions coming in - samples for testing - monitoring blood sugar going out as well as four IV's - protein, antibiotics, Zantac (prevent ulcers), Albumin (for the swelling) simultaneously sustaining her. Our own well being was on hold as we obsessed over her survival. What kept us going was hope. It was a tough fight - it was worth it - she was going to win.

Some said that Mom should not be given morphine for pain because she would become addicted to this narcotic. That would be the worst. The dictionary defines "worst" as "most ill" or "most painful." At this point there has been so much "ill" - so "much pain." Her present medication was about as effective as using a water pistol to put out a fire. The first day on heavy morphine left Mom barely conscious - unable to take nutrients in through a straw. The next day she was alert but in too much pain.

Nurse Jean had experience in pain management. Dr. Shikha and Jean came up with a balance to manage Mom's pain with percoset and morphine. Jean explained that Mom couldn't heal and suffer excruciating pain simultaneously. It made sense and gave us peace of mind that after days of hearing Mom cry, "God, help me," she would receive ongoing comfort to allow her body to heal itself from the surgery with God's power.

Jean said, "I hope you don't mind me giving my opinion." I thanked her and hugged her for educating us. We needed someone to reassure us that this is not a pain contest.

Dr. Friedman, Mom's gynecologist for eight years, removed the pessary holding the bladder in the hope it would bring electrolytes in the kidneys down.

I spoon fed Mom a small container of pudding; we want her off that I.V. and out of the hospital soon.

Peggy's father failed terribly during his last hospitalization. She felt, in retrospect, clear-cut goals for discharge might have produced a better outcome. Our dads socialized and went crabbing together thirty-five years ago. Our mothers did the church minstrel and mothers' guild as friends. We became friends at ages ten and eleven when my brother and her sister walked to school together.

My mother caught us arguing early in our friendship when I bragged to Peggy that since thirteen was the permissible age to wear lipstick I'd be a year ahead of her. Mom dried Peggy's tears telling me she felt that fourteen would be a better age for me to begin. That way Peggy and I could start together. Lipstick went out of style when we were thirteen and fourteen which we later joked about. My lesson was clear. If I behaved unkindly Mom would side against me. It spoke well of her integrity. She taught me how to embrace a lifelong friend like Peggy and, later, her husband, Ed. Peggy is a teacher. Ed is a high school principal. They are Bob and my reality checks on life. Ed's wry sense of humor could bring me to belly laughter even if I was in a depressed mood.

My mind is flooding with lifelong memories of my mother as a grandmother. John was here first - arriving in time to be embraced by my Dad who did not live long enough to see John graduate from the

University of Notre Dame. Mom cried when Kevin, at six years old, was hospitalized with bronchitis. She rejoiced when, as a naval officer, he had the honor to guide his ship into port at Newport, Rhode Island.

She laughed when young Michael decided he did not like chocolate. Mom prayed at Michael's daughter's christening four days after Michael escaped from Tower 2 of the World Trade Center.

Brian and Michael are Mets fans so they have an advantage with Mom over all of us. Mom cherishes the shadowy vision she sees when Brian holds his baby.

Danny's birth was a long process. I sat with Mom while I was nine months' pregnant with Jim while awaiting Danny's safe arrival. Bob had a card game going on at our house. When I called with the news they clapped, whistled, and cheered.

Neal held the rare distinction of being the fifth son to graduate from Christian Brothers Academy. During those years he helped Mom food shop where he worked part-time. He graduated from LaSalle University in December.

One of my children - my oldest, Jim - sometimes ran me ragged with hyperactivity. Mom told me that Jim would be successful.

109

He rejected schoolwork while devouring Time magazine. He does commodities contracts now five days a week while pursuing radio broadcasting on weekends.

Danielle is the grandchild who showed up at the nursing home to watch her grandmother lead the karaoke for the Christmas play. She's a financial analyst.

Todd, at six feet three inches tall just celebrated his twenty-first birthday this year. He's a Yankee fan and Mom will root with him only if the Mets lose.

Mom says she misses my Dad but is happy God allowed her to remain with us watching our families grow to share the good and the difficult into another generation.

I'm getting phone calls from her friends.Virginia sends Mom schedules of Met games written large and dark enough for Mom to decipher. I'm getting phone calls from Mr & Mrs. Croft and Mrs. Reilly, former neighbors who were there for Mom before my birth. Mrs. Croft lives in the same town as Mom's nursing home and visits her there. Mrs. Reilly celebrated her ninetieth birthday last year. Mr. & Mrs. Croft and Mom attended. Mom is not technology friendly and was quite impressed that Mrs. Reilly has a computer. Mom smiled when I said I was going to e-mail Mrs. Reilly. "I always knew that Mrs. Reilly was cool," I added.

The suffering of Good Friday continues into Holy Saturday when Mom is given drugs to ease her physical and mental pain. Rita Claire and I watch Mom constantly cough and our fear is pneumonia. When my brother-in-law, John, arrives at the hospital for his visit, he insists that Rita Claire and I leave. He tells us it is time for us to help ourselves because our anguish is apparent.

I call Dr. Shikha to express my concern. She promises to remedy the miscommunication. She had been scheduled to go to California that weekend. Instead, she told her husband that is not the right time for her to leave Rita Desmond. Her compassion brings me enormous strength when I need it most.

I returned in the evening and fed Mom ice cream. She was more alert, but looked sad. I told her that Danielle was at the mall picking up her new dress. "What color is the dress?" Mom asks. "Black," I answer.

Nurse Cathy assured me that Dr. Shikha's instructions for medication would be carefully followed. She said Mom's "God, help me" cries may be ICU psychosis from being imprisoned there too long. She gave me a supportive look when she saw my tear-stained face. She told me to try to have a nice Easter. I nodded and wished her the same.

The angel spoke, "Do not be frightened. I know you are looking for Jesus the crucified, but he is not here. He has been raised, exactly as he promised."

Matthew 28:5-6

The world with its difficulties continues. A Palestine suicide bomber victimizes Israel while my mother misses her Jewish dining companion. Race relations are unsettled at the time; Mom longs to be back in her home at the Bentley that is a room shared with an African-American friend.

We want Mom to be better. Her fate is out of our hands. Is there another problem the doctors are missing? Would the staff over-medicate because they are shorthanded? We gave no answers - only questions. Just like Mom, we wait and pray. My petition is "God, help her."

My Lord, I know what You are telling me
to watch the pain of those we love is harder
than to bear our own.
To carry my cross after You,
I, too, must stand and watch the sufferings of
my dear ones
the heartaches, sickness and grief of those I
love.

And I must let them watch mine too.

I do believe
for those who love You
All things work into good.

…Clarence Engler
Everyone's Way of the Cross

I tried not to behave like a lunatic when I arrived at the hospital on Easter Sunday at noon and Mom was still in bed. Her lungs stand a fighting chance in a chair. Her nurse,

Daryl, blows me off at first but is accommodating when I demand to see the floor supervisor. I explained to both of them that I am not looking to blame anyone. I'm frustrated because I want Mom to progress. I explain my feeling that overmedication was taking her out of the game. I told them I brought a radio because my son, Jim, will be a D.J. today on 106.3 F.M. from 2:00 p.m. to 7:00 p.m. but the antenna on the radio fell off. They get another radio and summon a team of four to move Mom to a chair. We tune in the radio. Linkin Park is playing "In the End." Daryl asks Mom if she wanted to dance. Then she gasps! Mom is moving her shoulders back and forth to the rhythm of the rock music. My mother is on her deathbed, yet she's dancing. This tells me there is still life in the old girl.

Loretta and Paul arrived for their Easter visit with Mom. I leave to finish dinner preparations. Todd had brought me a cooked meal for twenty from Wegman's. Jim is on the air now and I reminded Mom that even after Loretta and Paul leave she'll have Jim's voice to listen to between her naps. Danielle shared, "This is the first time that Grandma is not with us on a holiday. Yet, she is alive." I hug her and tell her I have hope.

I called the hospital at 6:15 p.m. to remind them that in about five or ten minutes Jim will reach out to his grandmother using the airwaves. You see, Rita Claire, Paul and I want to restrict visitors to our spouses and us.

Rita Claire, Paul and I with our families still gathered around our dining table listen as Jim speaks:

" I want to talk about the unrest in the world and hope for peace in Israel/Palestine. My grandmother has been in the hospital for a month. I know she's listening now. She has had four surgeries in the past month. I know I would find it difficult to have one and yet she had four. She claims her strength is faith in God and love for family and I want to tell her on behalf of our family that, "We love you, Grandma."

"Then he plays Creed's, "Higher."

Daryl called ten minutes later to say Mom heard every word of the dedication. They had the volume pumped up so that every worker, patient, and visitor who was not unconscious in ICU heard Jim tell Grandma, "We love you!"

"There are in the end three things that last: faith, hope, and love, and the greatest of these is love."

1 Corinthians 13:13

As the following week progressed, I became discouraged as I helplessly listened to my mother's relentless cough. Mom had pneumonia, a yeast infection and staph infection in the blood. My eyes filled with tears when I approached Dr. Arnold. I said, "She's not going to make it." Dr. Arnold put his arms around me, hugged me, and said, "She is going to make it. I'm going to explain why." He reached for a nearby computer and motioned for me to sit next to him on a chair with wheels as he pulled up her screen. He admitted the pneumonia was a concern and said that he agreed with me that getting her back to the Bentley's physical therapy team was advisable. It was her only chance.

"I have learned how to cope with every circumstance--how to eat well or go hungry, to be well provided for or do without. In him who is the source of my strength I have strength for everything."

Philippians 4:13

I have always been an Oprah fan. If I met her and she asked me what I know for sure I would say "I (Rita Claire and Paul) have a mother with a doctorate in Positive Attitude." This does not mean that she does not suffer or have negative feelings. It means she produces positive reactions despite what life throws at her.

We missed my dad on my wedding day, but it was joyful anyway. I met my husband on the anniversary of my dad's death and interpret that coincidence as God's gift to me. I was vacationing at the Jersey shore. Mom convinced me I should party with my young friends and not feel guilty she was widowed. That was such a selfless attitude; I hope to emulate it. Her social giftedness makes people-not just me-feel special and appreciated. In a busy world she always has time for everyone. Yet she repeatedly thanks me for spending time visiting and taking her to doctors. What she is oblivious to is that I am the recipient. Her presence is an ego trip for my soul. My sister, brother and me and our families are constantly blessed by the energy of her kind thoughts. Mom uses her mind to create happiness and we all have that ability. One of Mom's lowest moments was the realization that she would need to give up her apartment. Her coping strategy was thinking of others. She told Rita Claire and me to make a list of her belongings and which child or grandchild received the china or the table/chair set so that she could think about them getting pleasure from something belonging to her. "That will give me something nice to think about," she'd say. She laughed when I came to the Bentley last year wheeling her television in a garden wagon. I explained it was important that she watch the news. She said now she could watch the upcoming St. Patrick's Day parade.

125

The Mets were opening the 2001 baseball season and she was ready to cheer them on as she had since their conception, which was a few years before Mike Piazza, was born. She is not the fair weather fan who caught on with the successes of the last few years. She is the fan who stayed up until 2:00 a.m. listening to TV or radio when they were several games behind. If they even misplaced the roster they could have called Mom for the batting order and stats. What she does not know yet is that, while she was in surgery, Danielle and Jim were at a work seminar with Gary Carter and got their grandma a signed ball and picture from him. She will not be able to see it with her eyes, but she will see it with her heart. Our world is the beneficiary of Mom's simplicity and wisdom. We are still learning from her. I know that when God is ready for her she will fall into His loving arms and the devil knows he never stood a chance with her.

"It is only with the heart that one can see rightly. What is essential is invisible to the eye."

Antoine de Saint Exupery

Patricia Desmond Vargo

If the Mets win the World Series after that we will know it is because they deserve it and have the best fan possible rooting them on. The victory would come around the time we would have celebrated Aunt Ruth's 99th birthday.

God called Ruth home today. Our world was enriched by her ninety-eight years in this realm. One more thing I know for sure: Heaven is a better place today.

"Eye has not seen. Ear has not heard-what God has ready for those who love Him."

1 Corinthians 2:9-10

Somehow it all fell into place. Recovery was progressing and Mom was back in the game. Oh, there was work to do. She needed time to master those exercises. A month in bed took its toll, as it would on anyone. However, this time there was nothing holding her back. The clip was still there, but Dr. Arnold accommodated the stent to compensate for its presence. There was no gallstone obstruction, no multiple stones, no blood poisoning, no e-coli, no septic shock, no peritonitis, and no 40,000 white cell count. There was no blood clot that would get past, no ventilator, no four foot tube from the nose to the abdomen, no drains, no bandages to catch the "weeping" fluids trapped within, no roller coaster blood sugar of diabetes, no morphine stupor, no high or low blood pressure, no pessary, no kidney failure or elevated liver enzymes, no out of control heart arrhythmia. Let's not agonize over the latest internal bleeding episode because it stopped, but she had pneumonia.

We wanted her home. Home we visualized as the Bentley - with the roommate being Betty. Get to the hairdresser early Friday morning so you don't have to wait. How are her infant twins doing? Who is coming for happy hour on Friday afternoon? Did I hear that the Mets are on later? If so, we can talk up the strategy. Can we fit in a game or two of bingo before we line up for play?

If life were fair it would be reasonable for Mom to return to resume life as it had been for her - the poster lady for geriatrics at its best. My daughter, Danielle, helped me to see my folly saying, "Life is not always fair and you cannot expect these rewards just because Grandma suffered." We pray, we hope, we offer support, we accept.

I do not know what will be. Until I do I will visualize positive thoughts as my mother taught me. You see, that's my job as CEO of Rita Desmond - the lady standing at her Bentley court-view window watching the spring flowers bloom - maybe for the last time.

WHAT WILL YOU SAY ABOUT ME WHEN I AM GONE?

My cousin's wife, Natalie, died unexpectedly last spring at the young age of 60. Her two sons Rick and Merv gave a beautiful tribute of her life with them and her husband.

Later that day my mother asked me "What are you going to say about me?" I told her I would say she had the best attitude of anyone I know, which became the inspiration for a manuscript. Her cup was more than half full; it was overflowing.

My vision of my mother at this moment is as bright as the sun in Medjugorje, former Yugoslavia, with eighty years of receiving the Holy Eucharist illuminating her soul. Her face is many ages, reflecting only joyous peace. Her grandson, Daniel, has his arm around her and he towers above her height. My Dad is smiling letting her know she demonstrated courage for her remaining thirty-four years on earth without him.

My son Jim shared that when he saw Grandma suffering in the hospital his thoughts placed he and I thirty years into the future. In my mother he saw an older me as his empathy brought him into his 50's in my place. The suffering was difficult. Mom and I always repeated how we loved each other. I can honestly say to you at this moment: I did my very best. The remaining love is grace - my gift despite the former struggle.

I told Mom I would thank her for teaching Rita Claire, Paul, and I how to behave, respect ourselves, love, and accept God's will. She often told me, "Pat, stand up straight," and so I try not to slouch. Mom was proud of my passion and motivation. I admired her class and acceptance. In a busy world Mom always had time for everybody.

When I started kindergarten, I sat at the center table with seven other non-criers as the remainder of the class wailed. Many moms were grasping the window gate to see if their child was all right. I knew she would not be among them. Her expectation would be that I could survive without her physical presence.

Only my sister and brother know exactly how I feel. John, Loretta, and Bob valued Rita as a parent even though they brag about their bond in the "outlaw's club". All I know is that they always showed up for Mom and that our offspring gravitate to them.

Mom attended Pratt Business School and worked for the A&P main office when they were located in New York City so long ago. She retained a friendship with a lovely lady from that time named Connie, who moved to

135

Missouri. Although they never saw each other again they communicated over sixty years sharing joys and tragedy until Connie's death in the mid 90's.

Rita Claire planned Mom's 60th birthday. I planned Mom's 70th unaware that we wouldn't move into our new Marlboro home until two weeks before the party.

Paul and Loretta arranged dinner out with our Aunt Ruth and Mom for the last time they shared together. It was only a few months ago, but neither knew her fate. The logistics of that day defy belief with Ruth in Union, Mom in Jackson, a Sunday at the mercy of Route 9, dinner in Freehold and Paul and

Loretta in Ridgefield. Aunt Gert was recovering from back surgery at that time.

Mom told everybody I drove her to many doctor appointments, but she may not have shared she was my rock when Bob and I needed time away from raising a young family. Mom and I went to the American Hotel's "Oh Brothers" regularly for lunch. We always left each other replenished. In 1993 Mom accepted Rita Claire's idea and hosted a bridal luncheon there for her friend, Alice Cook, who married John at age 80.

My mother's love lives in me and within you because you are here today. I admired her simplicity, but only in her later years did I grow in wisdom to grasp how truly powerful she was. Every ounce of suffering you have felt comforting Gert, Rita Claire, Paul and I have served a purpose in God's good judgment.

I told Mom more recently that if we could document her attitude and teach it to others she could help others create happiness in their hearts and minds as she did. When her illness prevented her from attending the Bentley choir, she showed disappointment, "I waited all year for those Irish songs." My manager smiled when I told him "My mother is missing the Bentley. This is big! Most people dread nursing homes. My mother made it a happy experience because that was her choice.

My mother's legacy is: "We create our own happiness through our God, our families, our thoughts and how we treat others." This is her gift to me. This revelation is my gift to you.

"Mom, Rita, Grandma, Aunt Rita, Great Grandma, God must have spent a little more time on you. You are special. We will always love you!"

May the road rise to meet you.
May the wind be always at your back.
May the sun shine warm upon your face.
The rains fall soft upon your fields.
And, until we meet again,
May God hold you in the palm of His hand.
An Irish Blessing

"Pat, do you really think it is possible for me to see all my family at your house on Mother's Day?" Mom asked. I told her that was our new goal. The long awaited release from the hospital came on a Thursday. I felt spooked when she got her hair done the next day, which was a Friday - really early - so she didn't have to wait. The stylist's infant twins are thriving. The spring flowers were blossoming outside her court-view window just like they had in my visualization. However, what I had not considered was the toll Mom's mental attitude was subjected to by the trauma of all that had transpired. "Everyone's different, Pat. I'm different too."

I'll spare you the gory details until an incredible geriatric doctor created a plan to medicate my mother out of her hallucinations and paranoia of her reactive disorder. Intervention had to be here. I finally understood why the elderly fear hospitals.

Aunt Gert told me to pray to the Holy Spirit for the right words to tell of Ruth's passing. I know Gert's nightmare would be if her phone rang and my mother was on the other end saying, "Put Ruth on so I can speak to both of you." My nightmare was a well-meaning visitor saying, "I'm sorry you lost your sister." And Mom knowing she lost either Ruth or Gert. I told my mother that in order to get her out of the hospital when it happened it seemed

141

we needed one more person in heaven on our side-and that person is your sister - my Aunt Ruth. Mom cried, which was appropriate. She asked about the funeral and I told her how beautiful it was with our gratitude for Ruth's beautiful, faith-filled family focused on life. I assured her Gert was hanging in. A few days later I called Aunt Gert and they spoke briefly in a supportive way for the first time in seven weeks.

"Suddenly from up in the sky there came a noise like a strong, driving wind which was heard all through the house where they were seated. Tongues as of fire appeared, which parted and came to rest on each of them. All were filled with the Holy Spirit."

Acts 2:1-4

Mom did come to my house for Mother's Day. She didn't feel well, but spoke my favorite words, "Isn't it wonderful that we're all here together?"

When she returned to the hospital on her three-month deadline to have the clip opened, it was determined that the procedure was unnecessary. Apparently the clip mysteriously dislodged itself. There was no narrowing of the duct which was another pleasant surprise. She was then given a clean bill of health. Simultaneously, the announcement was made that former Met Gary Carter made the Hall of Fame.

Patricia Desmond Vargo

You gotta believe!

"Blest are they who have not seen and have believed."

John 20:29

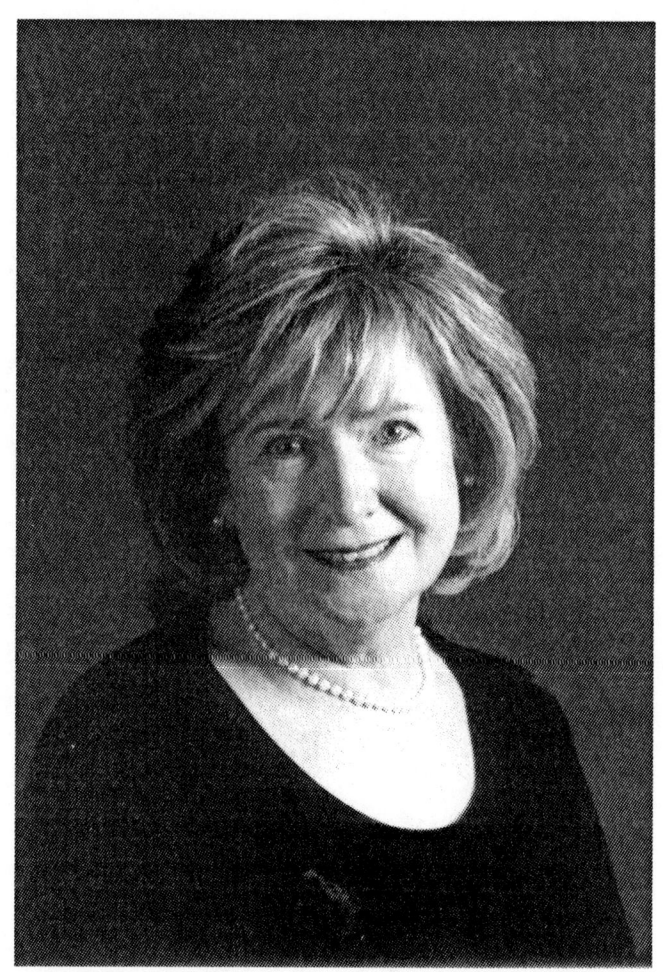

Patrica Vargo lives in Marlboro, NJ with her husband of 30 years Robert
and their adult children James, Danielle and Todd

Printed in the United States
1078500005B/331-378